I0420980

A Parent's Guide to Natural Therapies for Difficult & Challenging Behaviors (Including ADHD and Autism)

Amy E. Wicks, D.C.

Copyright © 2015 by Amy E. Wicks, D.C.
All rights reserved.

All rights reserved. No part of this publication may be
reproduced, distributed, or transmitted in any form or by any
means, including photocopying, recording, or other electronic
or mechanical methods, without the prior written permission
of the publisher, except in the case of brief quotations
embodied in critical reviews and certain other noncommercial
uses permitted by copyright law.

Printed in the United States of America
First Printing, 2015
Amy E. Wicks, D.C.
www.dramydc.com

ISBN: 1516823915
ISBN-13: 978-1516823918

Disclaimer
A Parent's Guide to Natural Therapies for Difficult &
Challenging Behaviors (Including ADHD and Autism) is not
intended as medical advice. This book is for educational and
informational purposes only. Always consult your medical
professional when the need arises. You are ultimately
responsible for the applications you make suggested in this
book.

About the Author

Amy Wicks, D.C., is a holistic chiropractor who focuses on using alternative methods of healing in order to treat the root cause of a problem. She graduated from Logan College of Chiropractic in St. Louis, Missouri, in 2012. She was the recipient of the Student Doctor Award given to one member of the graduating class. She is the owner and CEO of The Center for Natural Health, LLC, located in St. Charles, Missouri. She works with people of all ages who have learning disabilities, Autism Spectrum Disorder, and ADD/ADHD. She also helps with eczema, thyroid conditions, weight loss, digestive issues, food/environmental intolerances, and many more. She has incorporated chiropractic adjustments, nutrition, homeopathic remedies, acupuncture, essential oils, and the use of herbs into her practice. She is passionate about helping others learn natural ways to help with today's health concerns.

She has been happily married to her best friend since 2006 and has two biological sons and one stepson. She is a "hockey mom" and loves traveling with her family to all sorts of wonderful places. She is close to her parents, an older brother, and a younger sister. She loves the outdoors, sport activities, and spending time with her family. She is pictured on the cover with her youngest son.

This book is dedicated to all the parents who struggle with children who can be difficult and challenging. I hope this book inspires and encourages you to try a natural approach to help your children.

Table of Contents

Forward and Thanks

I am writing this book from the standpoint of a mom. My background has helped me with a lot of what I came up with along the way; however, it was the passion for my son that drove me to seek and find ways to help him without medication. I knew he was created for a purpose, but a lot of our toxic world was affecting his ability to live up to his true purpose. This book is written to help other parents who would like to be informed of some options to help their kids stay focused and maintain a healthy self-esteem without the use of medications.

I am a licensed chiropractor who works with "hard to treat conditions" with a thriving practice in St. Charles, Missouri. Many patients who knew I had a child who struggled with the symptoms of ADHD would ask how things were progressing with him. It came to the point that too much of the appointment time was focused on my son, rather than on the patient. It was then that I decided to write down everything I pursued and did, which is how this book was created. I truly hope this book is helpful for many families.

First, I would like to thank my husband for which all this would not be possible without his support. He has stood by me during my quest for natural therapies to help our family. I would also like to thank my mom for her continued support in helping my kids and for her desire for knowledge. Growing up, she always encouraged me to continue to learn and put the fire in me to seek more information. I would also like to thank my friend and colleague, Wendi Jones, D.C. She has been an inspiration to me. Without her, I would not have learned so much about the value of essential oils or how emotions can physically affect our bodies. I would like to thank Cheryl Colonello, M.D., who first introduced me to Isagenix and the value of quality protein for children. Last, but definitely not least, I would like to thank Amanda Thorne for introducing me to Juice Plus and allowing me to learn to become a better doctor by working with her and her wonderful children.

Why You Need to Read this Book

This book is about a natural approach for children who exhibit difficult and challenging behaviors. Some of these children have been given the diagnosis of ADD, ADHD, or Autism Spectrum Disorder; however, there are many who suffer from similar symptoms but don't have an actual diagnosis. These children might benefit from different therapies such as homeopathy, essential oils, NAET, nutrition, and more.

If you have been trying to figure out a way to help your child without medication or perhaps your child has no formal diagnosis but would still benefit from some natural therapies, please read this book. This book was created, designed, and written for parents like you!

A Parent's Guide to Natural Therapies

PART ONE

The Infant

Alex (who has been renamed for this book) was a beautiful, healthy bouncing baby boy born eight pounds and eight ounces. He nursed easily. He was calm and easy-going as an infant. He slept well and only awoke a couple times during the night. His older brothers loved holding him and helping out with him. It was truly a great first few months.

However, his first symptom actually appeared when he was just a few days old when he developed a clogged tear duct in his eye. This began a few short minutes after he was given the silver nitrate eye drops while at the hospital. The next symptom he had was continuously spitting up. These two symptoms were not enough for me to say, "Hey, something is wrong with my child"! These were very normal issues for an infant. I mean, the clogged tear duct isn't exactly normal, but his pediatrician wasn't worried, so I wasn't worried either. He was also breastfed which often creates more spit-up than formula.

The first four months were relatively easy. When he was four months, I began feeding him some baby food. We started with rice, and then added some vegetables. He stayed away from fruit at this point so he would develop a taste for vegetables. Unfortunately, every time he was fed, he would projectile vomit. I mean, it would literally leap across the room. This was not normal spit up. Besides, shouldn't food stay down more easily? After trying various foods with the same result, I became concerned. The only food he was able to keep down was green peas. At this point, I believed it warranted a visit to his pediatrician. Perhaps something was wrong with his lower esophageal sphincter which is designed to hold food in the stomach. It's common for that sphincter to be still developing in infants.

After a visit with his pediatrician, we discovered that nothing was wrong with his esophageal sphincter. I was given instructions to keep feeding him the different foods. He would eventually be able to keep them down. I was extremely unhappy with this answer because I knew something was wrong. It was almost like he was allergic to everything I fed him.

MY AH-HA!

That's when I had my first "light-bulb" moment, my AH-HA! I remembered many years back when I was an office manager for a chiropractor who did some desensitization treatments for different foods. That day, I got on the phone and made an appointment for Alex. It was a 45 minute drive one way, and the cost was a little high since she did not take insurance, but I was willing to try anything. Currently, I was changing his clothes as well as mine three to four times a day. I had had enough. If I only gave him breast milk, he was cranky and hungry and didn't sleep well. I also didn't want to feed him peas the rest of his life.

After the first visit with the holistic chiropractor, we discovered that Alex was "reacting" to many foods. He was even reacting to my breast milk, which explained why he was constantly spitting up the breast milk. We began desensitization treatments that day (breast milk being the first), and he slowly began to improve. I was able to increase his food choices as we progressed with his treatments, and life began to get easier.

NAET

The desensitization technique the holistic chiropractor used is called NAET, Nambudripad Allergy Elimination Technique. It's a wonderful technique, and I use it in my office today. NAET is a non-invasive, drug free, natural solution to alleviate allergies of all types and intensities using a blend of selective energy balancing, testing and treatment procedures from acupuncture, acupressure, allopathy, chiropractic, nutritional, and kinesiological disciplines of medicine. (For further information on NAET, see Appendix B or visit www.naet.com.)

At six months of age, just a couple months after we began NAET protocol, I took him for his sixth month baby well visit. At this time, he wasn't doing some of the things on the sheet that were age appropriate for a six month old. I was concerned about it and asked his pediatrician. He said he wasn't concerned, and he seemed to be doing fine. I innocently agreed with him because he said that my older son was just ahead of the curve, so it seemed like Alex was a little delayed. I know parents aren't supposed to compare kids, but when you have your first child you are typically oblivious to what the standard learning curve is, so you tend to gauge your other children on what the older one does. I have since gotten away from that because I realize that both my boys are extremely different and wonderful in their own way and need their own style of parenting.

THERE HE WAS!

A month after his sixth month well visit, and three months after beginning NAET protocol, I noticed something different about Alex. I noticed that he would look at me more, but it was more than just looking at me. It was like he didn't have a glaze over his eyes. This part is hard for me to explain, but I'm sure some parents out there will be able to relate. The first seven months of his life he would occasionally look at people, but it was like there was no one inside. I didn't even realize that's what it was until the day he looked at me, and THERE HE WAS! It was like he was registering everything he was seeing. He seemed to have finally come into his own body, and a fog had been lifted. His speech began to pick up, and many of his motor skills began to develop much better than they were.

At 12 months, we had an appointment scheduled with a pediatric ophthalmologist for surgery on his tear duct. It still remained clogged from the second day in the hospital. We prayed that he wouldn't need surgery and continued with the NAET protocol to try and clear up the tear duct. Two days before his appointment, the tear duct opened and tears began draining appropriately into the nasal cavity. We kept the appointment just to be sure everything was healed, and it was.

MY DECISION TO SUPPORT RECOVERY

We continued NAET protocol until he was around 15 months of age, which is when I decided to go back to school to become a chiropractor. NAET was an overriding factor in my decision to return to school to become a chiropractor. The changes I saw in Alex after the NAET protocol is what made the decision final. I thought about becoming a chiropractor in the past because NAET helped my own environmental allergies, but the improvement in Alex is what made me take the leap.

What fascinated me the most about NAET is how it revealed to me so many things that I didn't know. A person doesn't know what they don't know. My eyes were opened to many more possibilities. Some of the NAET protocol consists of treating the person for vitamin C and B vitamins. How can someone be "reacting" to these things? Our bodies need these to survive so how can you react to it? Sometimes the body doesn't use the vitamins or minerals the way it was designed.

NAET allows the body to use proper nutrients. When the body is able to use what it needs, recovery can begin.

What did I learn in this chapter?

- Foods truly can play a role in our physical health and mental health.
- NAET did some amazing work with Alex.
- Every child is unique and must be treated as a unique individual.
- Alternative Therapies really can help.

PART TWO
The Toddler

During Alex's toddler years (ages two - three), I was a full time student at Logan College of Chiropractic, and Alex was at home with my mom. He was an active child, to say the least. He constantly needed to be active. So, we let him be active. He is the youngest of three boys. When Alex was two, his brothers were 14 and six. Both brothers are his half-brothers, and his oldest brother has mild autism (the 14 year-old is my stepson and the six year-old is my biological son; both older boys are from previous relationships). We have a very active home.

HOW MUCH SLEEP DO CHILDREN NEED?

Even with Alex being active all day, he was still having some trouble with sleep. He had trouble falling asleep at night, and then once he fell asleep, he wouldn't stay asleep. This was frustrating because he wasn't getting the amount of sleep he needed, and then he was an even more rambunctious child during the day. I was also frustrated because I was in the middle of a full college class load (30+ credit hours). It became difficult for me to study and learn what I needed to learn in order to perform well in school, but I got through it. I decided I needed to stay at school a little longer at the end of the day in order to study and finish homework.

We had to do away with naps altogether at the age of two because if he had a nap, he would not fall asleep at night until after 11:00 pm. That did not work for me since I had to be up at 5:30 a.m. for school, and my husband had to be at work usually by 4:00 a.m.

The importance of sleep cannot be over estimated. That is the time for the body to repair itself, including the brain and nervous system. When a child does not get enough sleep, or good quality sleep, it often will result in hyperactivity during the day.

Studies suggest that about 25 percent of children do not get enough sleep.**

The following indicates the average total amount of sleep children need at various ages.

- 1 yr old = 11.75 hours (includes 2 naps)
- 2 yr old = 11.5 hours (includes 1 nap)
- 3 yr old = 11.25 hours (includes 1 nap)
- 4 yr old = 11 hours
- 5 yr old = 10.75 hours
- 6 yr old = 10.5 hours
- 7 yr old = 10.5 hours
- 8 yr old = 10.25 hours
- 9 yr old = 10 hours
- 10 yr old = 10 hours
- 11 yr old = 9.75 hours
- 12 yr old = 9.5 hours
- 13 yr old = 9.25 hours
- 14 yr old = 9.5 hours
- 15 yr old = 9.25 hours
- 16 yr old = 9 hours
- 17 yr old = 9 hours
- 18 yr old = 9 hours

The information in the chart was taken from Ferber, Richard. *Solve Your Child's Sleep Problems. (pp. 10-11). New York: Fireside Book, 2006.***

SUGGESTIONS FOR SLEEP

- Bedtime Routine - Allow child to "wind down."
- Epsom Salt Baths - Good for relaxing especially if you combine it with lavender oil or chamomilla oil.
- Homeopathic Remedies - Chamomilla helps calm down the nervous system as well as Ignatia Amara.
- Read a story before bed.
- White noise in the background can help - fan, white noise maker, calming music.
- Salt lamp - Air purifier, aids in sleep and can double as a night light.
- Essential Oils - Peace and Calming, Lavender, or Chamomilla

HOMEOPATHIC REMEDIES

It was during this time that I learned a lot about homeopathic remedies. Homeopathic remedies are diluted concentrations of an actual substance. The idea is that "like cures like." For example, the homeopathic remedy Belladonna comes from the belladonna plant and is used in a highly diluted quantity. For more detailed information on homeopathic remedies see Appendix A.

We began giving Alex Belladonna, Ignatia Amara and Chamomilla to help with his sleep and some behavioral problems. All three helped with his sleep as well as behavior. We gave Alex his homeopathic remedies, usually 12x dosage, at bedtime as well as in the morning before school. Most homeopathic remedies come in the form of dissolvable tablets, but some can be liquid drops. I often use a dosage of 12x with Alex, however; sometimes I will use a 30x. I suggest seeing a homeopathic doctor to get correct remedy and dosing.

A brief explanation of the homeopathic remedies we used is listed below. Dosages are not provided as each child is different, and proper dosages should be discussed between the doctor and the parent.

Belladonna is great for someone who has trouble learning, has sensitivity to noise and light, tends to be forgetful, has night terrors, has a fear of ghosts, and/or complains of hot and throbbing discomfort. Belladonna helps bring these in balance.

Ignatia Amara is good for someone who expresses strong emotions. It helps with insomnia, worry, depression, sadness, anger, mental and physical exhaustion, as well as hiccups and headaches.

Chamomilla helps with irritability, impatience, complaining, frustration, restless, and bad tempers. A person who benefits from chamomilla is someone who demands one thing and then wants something else; quiets down once he has attracted attention; whines and screams; and likes to be carried, jiggled or rocked. He has (or may have) an aversion to being touched with a hypersensitivity to pain. Symptoms tend to be worse at night.

There are other homeopathic remedies that have been shown to help with ADHD, but these are the three I found helpful. In December 2005, the *European Journal of Pediatrics* published two studies. The first was a clinical observation study followed by a randomized, double blind, placebo controlled crossover trial. A crossover trial means that half of the patients begin with a placebo treatment, while the other half begin with homeopathy. After six weeks, the "crossover" occurs, and the groups each receive the other treatment. The two studies concluded that homeopathy has positive effects in patients with attention deficit hyperactivity disorder (ADHD). The crossover trial suggests scientific evidence of the effectiveness of homeopathy in the treatment of attention deficit hyperactivity disorder, particularly in the areas of behavioral and cognitive functions (Frei, Everts, von Ammon, *et al.*, 2005).

The challenge with homeopathic remedies is

finding the correct one that matches your child. Below is a list of some homeopathic remedies that have been helpful for difficult and challenging children. One remedy may be enough for your child, but in my experience using two to three has more of an impact. Please see the following for more information as to what symptoms it may be able to help.

- **Stramonium** - Children with many fears might benefit from Stramonium.
- **Cina** – Children who can be physically aggressive might benefit from Cina.
- **Hyoscyamus Niger** – Children with manic symptoms might benefit from Hyoscyamus Niger.
- **Tarentula Hispana** – Children who tend to be mischievous, sneaky, wild and crazy, worse with music, feels insulted, hurried, restless, frenzied might benefit from Tarentula Hispana.
- **Verta Alb** – Children who are hyperactive and need to be calmed might benefit from Verta Alb.
- **Hyoscyamus** – Children who are restlessness and hyperactive might benefit from hyoscyamus.
- **Tuberculinum** – Children who are very restless and seek constant stimulation may benefit from Tuberculinum.
- **Arsen lod** – Children who have emotional

outbursts and temper tantrums might benefit from Arsen lod.

DEVELOPMENTAL MILESTONES

Developmentally, at age two, Alex still would not make direct eye contact for more than two or three seconds. When he was told, "Look at me" he would respond with "I am," but his eyes were always looking off in the distance. When we would try to take his picture, it was a rare occasion for us to be able to get him to look at the camera. In most of his pictures, his eyes are all over the place.

On the other hand, his large motor skills were developing extraordinarily well, but he still struggled with fine motor skills. He wasn't able to hold a crayon correctly. His drawings and colorings were developmentally behind. His speech, however, was progressing. He had a large range of vocabulary, but his words would often be slurred. He struggled with pronouncing some of the alphabet. We had him tested for speech through our public school district, but he didn't have enough of a delay to warrant help through the school district. The speech therapist who tested him said he had a 34% delay, and he had to be at 50% or greater to warrant aid through the district.

FEARS

The greatest issue we faced during Alex's toddler years was his development of multiple fears. It's typical for some fears to develop in the toddler years, but his fears were extreme. He wanted his main overhead light on all night as he slept. Having any kind of light on during sleep is not conducive to good quality sleep. We compromised with two night lights in the room. He wanted the closets closed all the way, two night lights on, sometimes three, the radio playing with classical music, a fan blowing, and a stuffed animal. It seemed obsessive, but we did it because if it helped him fall asleep and stay asleep, we were willing to try anything.

When it comes to sleep, your brain needs complete darkness in order to produce enough melatonin. Melatonin is the sleep-inducing hormone that causes your body to fall asleep and stay asleep. Even artificial light after dark can send messages to the brain telling it to wake-up. According to a peer reviewed research article published in PLOS ONE, the selection of commercially available compact fluorescent lights with different colour temperatures significantly impacts on circadian physiology and cognitive performance at home and in the workplace (Chellappa SL, Steiner R, Blattner P, Oelhafen P, Götz T, et al.). I was in a "Catch-22." He was so scared to fall asleep without a lot of light, but then if I had the light on, his brain wouldn't produce the hormone he needed in order to fall asleep and stay asleep. He continued to wake up at least once throughout the night during his toddler years.

We learned a lot about the importance of sleep during the toddler years. We also learned how homeopathic remedies can help with many behaviors as well as sleep. The next chapter will discuss some educational behavioral issues we encountered, differences in children's learning ability, and the importance of great teachers.

What did I learn in this chapter?

- Homeopathic remedies can help difficult and challenging children.
- Homeopathic remedies can help with sleep and behavioral issues.
- A proper amount of sleep is extremely important for optimal child development.
- Emotions can play a role in children's sleep patterns.

PART THREE

The Preschooler

At age three, Alex began attending preschool. The first couple months went smoothly. He, of course, was scared to attend the first few days, but he quickly became accustomed to the routine and fell right in place. We had Alex signed up for only two half days a week, because we weren't quite sure how he would adjust to the program.

After Alex was in preschool for several weeks, I went to pick him up and he was not in his classroom. I was informed that he was in the principal's office due to a behavioral problem. I thought to myself, "Oh boy. Here we go. What could he possibly have done that warranted a visit to the principal's office?" I felt like I was the one in trouble as I walked down the hallway. I was always the rule follower, the good kid in school. Not once did I have detention, let alone have to go to the principal's office, and now I was on my way there for my three-year-old son.

It turns out that he was swinging his book-bag in the hallway. He was told numerous times to stop, but he did not listen or heed the warnings. The book-bag was taken away from him due to his continued swinging. Now, the book-bag is not the reason he was sent to the office. It's what came after that sent him down the hall to the office. When the book-bag was taken away, he fell down on the ground and began kicking and waving his arms, screaming at the top of his lungs, and hitting and kicking anyone who came near him. He basically had a complete "meltdown." They weren't sure what happened or what to do with him.

COULD IT BE AUTISM?

After Alex's meltdown at school, we had a flashback of similar behavior from his half-brother. Alex's half brother, my stepson, was diagnosed with mild autism around the age of three. I also did a project on Autism during a postgraduate course I took (prior to meeting my husband). Now, obviously, my son Alex did not have all the signs and symptoms of someone with Autism Spectrum Disorder. However, due to his somewhat delayed progress developmentally, his lack of eye contact, and now a major behavioral incident in the school hallway, I feared autism. I called the chiropractor who performed the NAET treatments on him a year and a half earlier and asked her what her thoughts were. She suggested I bring him in.

We took him in to have him checked for the NAET Autism Protocol, which is very effective in treating the symptoms associated with autism. He was a candidate for the protocol. This does not in any way diagnose him as having autism, but it gave us a route to proceed with proper NAET treatments to help stimulate his brain in the appropriate way. I wanted this to be done as soon as possible, as I was fully aware how quickly his brain was developing. Brain development begins to slow down around age three, but still continues at a very high pace until the age of seven where brain development takes another dip and slows some more. Our brains are continually developing over the course of our life, but the rate at which they develop decreases as we age. This is known as neuroplasticity - *neuro means nerve and plasticity means flexible*. Therefore the brain has the ability to create new neurological (nerve) pathways or synapses (connections) due to thinking, emotions, behavior, environment, injury, or neural processes.

FINANCIAL COMMITMENT

I wanted Alex to have as many NAET treatments as possible in order to help his brain create the appropriate neurological pathways during high developmental stages. Since we had already done all the basic NAET treatments when he was younger, we were able to move straight to some NAET treatments to help with neurological development. We decided to take him three times a week to complete as quickly as possible. It took a good amount of commitment from my husband and me since this was all out of pocket expense, not covered by insurance, and the office was 45 minutes each way. My husband was working 60 hours or more a week, and I was in school full time with over 30 credit hours. We still had a total of three kids to take care of, one very active in sports. Needless to say, we were exhausted and financially tight (as I was not working), but God provided a way for it to happen. This is also where I give a big shout-out to my mom for always being there for me. When we needed her to take Alex to the doctor, she would take him. She watched Alex during the day when he wasn't in school. She came to our house at 5:30 every morning, got the kids ready for school, drove them to school and then picked them up from school. She did all of it for free and without complaining. She also continued to work at her full time job. My mom is truly a Godsend and I will forever love and appreciate her. Thank you, Mom.

SCHOOL INCIDENTS

We started to notice some behavioral changes, but they didn't happen overnight. There was another incident at school when Alex decided to pull down his pants in the classroom. This was done in total innocence, but nonetheless, it required a phone call home. We explained to him that it isn't appropriate to show anyone his penis, but he didn't understand why. We had to leave it at "just don't do it." Alex did better for the rest of the year, but he still continued to have some behavioral problems.

I decided to attend the Christmas party they had at Alex's school the last day before winter break. It was during this time I noticed that Alex seemed to understand the directions better than the other kids in his class. The children were instructed to sit in a circle, and while the music was playing they were to pass the presents to the person to their right. Most three-year-olds don't know which way is right. Basically, they played hot potato with presents. The music came on, and Alex went right to what he was instructed to do. Only one other child in the circle knew what to do. Alex was doing his best to explain to the other kids not to hold onto the present until the music stopped and that they had to keep passing it until the music stopped. He was getting very frustrated because the kids just kept trying to hold the presents or pass them in the wrong direction. I could see he was about to have a fit, when the music stopped, and he received a present to open.

LIGHT BULB MOMENT

Could his behavioral problems be due to the fact he was bored at school and learning things faster than the other kids? Every child is great and unique in his or her own right. However, children learn differently, and some kids do learn more quickly than others, which can create some behavioral issues.

We were suspicious that Alex was a strong kinesthetic learner (learns through movement), which can sometimes give the illusion of ADHD. The Director of the National Reading Diagnostics Institute, Ricki Linksman, M.ED., informs us that many children are given the diagnosis of Attention Deficit Hyperactivity Disorder, but in-depth reading evaluations show they are simply kinesthetic learners rather than having an attention disorder. When these children have the *"opportunity to learn through proper methods, their*

ADHD-like behavior often disappears" (Linksman, 1999).

KINESTHETIC LEARNERS

Kinesthetic learners prefer to move around, explore, and use their muscles for optimal results. A few examples of kinesthetic learning methods are writing in sand or shaving cream, using a flashlight to write, or walking while studying. These students can face frustration when they are asked to sit and be still for long periods of time. Many times, these students will get up often to sharpen their pencils, use the restroom, or drops things just so they can move to pick up the item. They may volunteer to run errands for teachers or be class monitors. If they are unable to perform in any of these activities, they often will begin wiggling in their seats, tapping their pencil, rocking, or leaning back in chairs. If you would like to know if your child is a kinesthetic learner, Ricki Linksman, M.ED., has created an online test to help you determine your child's fastest way of learning. This test can be found at the following link, www.superlinkslearning.com.

THE END OF THE SCHOOL YEAR

During the rest of the year, Alex continued to improve, but he remained extremely active in school and at home. At school when they had their end of the year assembly, all the kids were up on stage performing and singing. My child was the one on the end waving his hand at me, yelling "Hi" numerous times, and dancing to his own beat, while all the other kids were standing nicely and appropriately. He was very comical though, and I loved every minute of that assembly. Thank goodness I have it recorded so I can watch it over and over again. You can just see his personality shining through!

THE BEST TYPE OF SCHOOL FOR ALEX

Towards the end of the year, my husband and I contemplated where to put him for preschool the following year. He didn't seem to be learning anything at the school he was attending. He still didn't know all his colors, could only count to three, and his fine motor skills were still delayed. We were discussing a Montessori school because from what we could tell, it helps to develop kids based on their own personal skill level. We felt this would be a good fit for him as it seemed to focus more on a one-to-one approach of learning. A few weeks before the end of school, we received a phone call from his teacher. She wanted to discuss another incident that happened at school. During the course of the conversation, she mentioned that she did not think that his current school would be a good fit for Alex next year. She reiterated how much she loved the school and even sent her daughter there, but the four-year-old class had 24 students. Alex currently only had 10 students in his classroom and was continually having distraction problems. She said he struggled with focusing on any tasks at hand and was afraid he would struggle even more with that many kids in the classroom. I agreed and asked her what her thoughts were on a Montessori program for him. She agreed she thought he would do well in that type of program. So, we found a local Montessori school and enrolled him on a part time basis. We started him in the summer so that he would have time to get used to the new school before the actual preschool program began since Alex has struggled with changes since he was a baby.

This was another huge financial commitment from us, as Montessori schools tend to cost quite a bit. We decided it was worth a try.

The next chapter will discuss the Montessori chapter of Alex's life. A lot happened while he was four and five, so much that it deserves its own chapter.

What did I learn in this chapter?

- NAET treatments can help with cognitive function.
- Brain development is continuous throughout our lives, but slows as we age.
- Boredom at school can create behavioral issues.
- Kids who learn faster need as much assistance as kids who have some learning difficulties.
- Kinesthetic learners can sometimes mimic Attention Deficit Hyperactivity Disorder.

PART FOUR

Our Montessori Years

At the age of four, Alex needed a different school experience. The summer after his fourth birthday, which was in May, he began going to a Montessori preschool. The teachers were wonderful, and the staff was amazing. We decided to enroll him during the summer so he would have a chance to warm up to the new school, the new teacher, and the new kids. When preschool began, we wanted to be certain that he was able to learn without any distractions of "newness."

That summer was amazing! Our little four-year-old began counting to ten within just a few short weeks. He knew all his colors shortly thereafter. He loved going to school every day. This was also the summer he actually taught himself how to swim and swing on the swing-set. All this he learned while attending the Montessori school. His accomplishments reiterated to us that he was indeed a strong kinesthetic learner. The children went swimming every Thursday where he learned to swim. They had the swing-sets outside where he was able to practice every day. On nice days, the kids would stay outside almost all day. With the Montessori Method, learning is done everywhere and anywhere.

PRESCHOOL BEGINS

When the fall rolled around, it was time to begin actual preschool and true Montessori learning. His learning continued at a phenomenal rate, and we were very pleased. I think the biggest difference we noticed in our son was his self-esteem. We couldn't believe how much his self-esteem was increasing. In September, the school had their annual meeting for the parents where we were able to see the classroom, meet the teachers, other parents, and go over classroom expectations. They also discussed the Montessori Method, good for us since we didn't know anything about how it differed from the regular teaching method. We were told to let Alex do almost everything on his own. He had to make sure he dressed himself every day, picked out his own clothes, brushed his teeth, combed his hair, etc. We also needed to make sure he was able to reach all of his own clothes. When I heard this, my first thought was, "Are you kidding me? There is no way my child will do ANY of that on his own!" Well, since we decided to be all-in, we reconstructed his closet (okay, my husband did as I am not very handy with shelving) so all his clothes would be at his height.

The next morning after we moved all of his clothes to a lower, appropriate level for him, he was up and dressed before I was even out of bed! I then asked him if he brushed his teeth. He replied NO and then asked if I would show him how. Absolutely! was my response. He has been getting his own clothes out and dressing himself completely ever since. I will admit there are some days I cringe and bite my tongue when the outfits he chooses do not match, such as a nice polo collared shirt with camouflage sweat pants. However, we made a deal that if we had to go somewhere nice, such as church, I was allowed to veto an outfit if it wasn't appropriate. This agreement has worked since.

DOES FOOD REALLY PLAY A ROLE?

This is the year I began doing research with food and certain diets to help with behavior, hyperactivity, and learning disabilities. I decided to do a hair analysis (today I would opt for blood work as the hair analysis was done in Europe and their food differs from ours) which showed if he was allergic and/or sensitive to any foods or airborne particles in the environment like grass, pollen, mold, etc. Of course, the analysis came back listing too many for us to avoid. We decided to have him avoid wheat/gluten and corn as those were his greatest sensitivities. This seemed to help a bit, but not drastically. I would also like to point out that the school was amazing at accommodating our requests to have only gluten free foods and corn free foods. We, of course, had to bring in some gluten free bread for occasions the meal that was prepared had some wheat in it, which we were happy to do. A lot of schools will not accommodate in any way, so we were blessed to be at a school that would.

We followed the gluten free and corn free diet for about seven months. We decided to allow those back into his diet as we didn't see much of a difference. Keep in mind that we had already "cleared" or treated wheat, gluten and corn with the NAET protocol, which to me would explain why we didn't see much of a change by going gluten free and corn free. His body had already figured out how to manage those sensitivities and intolerances due to the NAET work that was done earlier. I believe the hair analysis revealed these sensitivities because the food in Europe is different than our food in America. A lot of food in America is made from Genetically Modified Organisms (GMOs). Many nations in Europe have banned GMOs.

Even though we didn't see much of a change with the gluten free and corn free diet, we did notice a change in his behavior with sugary foods and artificial additives. *The American Journal of Psychiatry* published a systemic review and meta-analysis that concluded, *"Free fatty acid supplementation produced small but significant reductions in ADHD symptoms even with probably blinded assessments... Artificial food color exclusion produced larger effects but often in individuals selected for food sensitivities"* (Catalá-López, Ferrán et al., 2015). We began cooking with coconut oil regularly to help increase his fatty acid content. Keeping Alex away from sugary foods and artificial additives is much more difficult. Even when we tried to keep him away at home, he still got some of it at school or at a friend's house. It took a few days for his system to "wind-down" after having had too much sugar or artificial additives.

NEUROTRANSMITTERS

The school year ended, and we had to decide if we were going to continue with the Montessori school for kindergarten or enroll him in their sister school where my older son attended. This was actually a very difficult decision. The Montessori school was going through some restructuring. Every single teacher was going to be a new hire, and all the current teachers were being let go. I'm not sure of the politics why this was happening, as to nor did I really want to get into the middle of the situation. After a lot of deliberation and consideration, we decided to continue Alex at the Montessori school. We were afraid that he wasn't mature enough for a regular kindergarten classroom. We decided that if he wasn't performing well in kindergarten at the Montessori school, we would then re-enroll him in kindergarten at the sister school the following year.

Over the summer between preschool and kindergarten, I did a lot of "work" with him. We focused a little on actual school work, but mostly my focus was on getting him to pay attention and focus. I remember learning about neurotransmitter sprays from a seminar I had taken a couple years back. Neurotransmitter testing can be performed through a simple urine or saliva test. I use Pharmasan Labs from NeuroScience, Inc. in my office.

He did end up needing a spray called Acetyl-flow, which is comprised of ingredients the brain needs to create acetylcholine. Acetylcholine is one neurotransmitter used for learning. Sometimes, kids with learning difficulties or ADD/ADHD have too many neurotransmitters or too little. In Alex's case, he had too little and needed some extra acetylcholine. He also needed to take a homeopathic remedy (Neurotrans Active) that was comprised of 4 different major neurotransmitters: Acetylcholine, GABA, Serotonin, and Dopamine. I gave him a couple sprays of acetylcholine called Acetyl-flow and a couple sprays of the Neurotrans-Active every morning before school.

BEHAVIORAL PROBLEMS

When school began, I also started him on Belladonna and Ignatia Amara. Both are great homeopathic remedies that I have found to be helpful with some of the behavior problems associated with autism and ADD/ADHD. The first few months of kindergarten went well. However, around November, we started getting negative remarks about Alex from his teachers. Teachers remarked that Alex was exhibiting these behaviors: name-calling, kicking, punching, disrespect, lack of interest in school, etc. "Here we go again," I thought to myself. What I couldn't wrap my head around is why he did so well the year before and then BAM! right back to where we left off at the other preschool. What was going on?

We were having behavioral issues at home as well. He hated school. He never wanted to go in the mornings. He would call himself stupid and say he couldn't do anything. As a mom, this really broke my heart and frustrated me at the same time. How can my five-year-old be saying these things? I needed to know if there was something I could be doing further at home to help with his self esteem, or was something going on at his school that was affecting him so deeply?

We had a teacher conference after he hit another boy. The director didn't say Alex was being kicked out, but she made it clear they were considering that option. I, of course, was also concerned why my child became so disruptive in class, refusing to do the work, and hitting other kids. Granted, he does have an older brother whom he wrestles with all the time (as well as his dad), but he knew not to do it at school. Since I was at my wits' end and concerned for my son, I made an appointment for him to see a well-respected child psychologist in the area.

CHILD PSYCHOLOGIST

The child psychologist talked with him for a while, asked him some questions, and then sent him to "the other side of the window" so she could speak to my husband and me without him hearing. She informed us that he was extremely smart (my husband and I looked at each other at this point with big eyes, as if saying to each other "Really? Are you sure?" We love Alex, but that one didn't cross our minds). We questioned her at that remark, and she reiterated that he was, then continued on saying that he seemed to be very stubborn (Ummmm...yes, nailed that one). We felt that he was smart, but at other times we felt like he had a great learning disability. He would go back and forth on his progress in school and constantly tell us that he didn't understand something. He would also say "I forgot" constantly. He made comments at times of misbehavior that "my brain is bothering me."

She went on to say that when you get someone as intelligent as he is and stubborn at the same time, you tend to get a manipulative and lazy child. Holy Cow, that was Alex! If he didn't want to do something, he always found a way out of it. She also stated that he had an excellent memory. Again, that surprised us since he was always saying he forgot something. She said that he was borderline ADHD, but she didn't want to give him that actual diagnosis yet since he was only five years old. I agreed. She also stated that with his personality, he would not do well in a Montessori school. He needed to have structure, consequences for misbehavior, but more importantly, he needed positive rewards for appropriate behavior. Alex needed someone to tell him what to work on or he wouldn't do it. He would choose the easier tasks that he had already mastered instead of choosing tasks that challenged him. This was very different from what we were used to with our parenting skills. We had to change it up a bit for him.

CAUGHT IN THE ACT

When we got home that day, I asked Alex if he did something (I can't remember what it was now, but what followed I remember very well). His response, as he was jumping on and off the couch, was "I forgot." I immediately responded, "The doctor just told us you have an excellent memory, so please stop telling me you forgot something." His reaction is burned into my memory forever. As soon as those words came out of my mouth, he stopped jumping around, looked at me directly in the eyes as if he were shooting daggers at me. He then went and did whatever it was I asked him to do. We rarely heard the words "I forgot" again. Sorry Alex, but the cat is out of the bag! I realized that day that he had been manipulating us, his parents, into thinking he couldn't do stuff. Now, there are some things that he truly does struggle with, at which point we help him. However, we have been able to better determine when he really needs help and when he just doesn't feel like doing something. One way we try to differentiate if Alex truly needs help is asking him if he really needs help or if he just doesn't want to do it. It helps if it's a task I know he can do or has done in the past; then I can differentiate if he needs help or wants help. I encourage him to clarify his needs and wants. To determine what he needs help with and what he wants help with demands getting to know Alex: his demeanor, his attitude, his facial expressions. I had to study his expressions when I knew he wasn't being fully honest as well as when he was being honest. That is still and probably will always be a work in progress. Listed below are some strategies you can use with your child which is good for both parents and teachers alike:

- Ask your child if he/she really NEEDS help or if he/she just doesn't want to do the task at hand.

- Study your child's body language, including facial expressions, to determine if your child is being honest or dishonest.

- Encourage your child to clarify their needs

versus their wants.

ACETYLCHOLINE

In all the chaos, I realized that I had stopped giving him the Acetyl-flow neurotransmitter spray. I had run out and not remembered to order more. Quite honestly, I didn't see the importance of it since he was doing well at the beginning of school. Things were going well, and I didn't make the connection that a lot of his behavior and struggles at school developed shortly after we stopped the neurotransmitter sprays. I immediately ordered more. We began the sprays as soon as they arrived, but I knew it would take at least a week, or longer, before his system would have enough to function properly. Acetylcholine is often given to children to increase learning. So, when a child is in school, they are sucking up that neurotransmitter like it's going out of style. I basically had to "fill up his tank" so to speak.

SALT BATHS

At this time, I also began using therapeutic grade essential oils mixed with some Epsom Salt. He would have this in his bath every night before bed along with a very strict routine. The salt baths helped more than I had anticipated or expected. They would calm him down immediately. I remember the first time I used a salt bath for Alex. He was inconsolable and crying. Neither his dad nor I were able to calm him down. After about half an hour of him crying, I remembered the bath salts mixed with different essential oils I had gotten as a Christmas gift from a colleague. I started the bath and added "Believe" salt bath. I poured it in and mixed it around to dissolve. Alex stepped in (still crying) and about 30 seconds after sitting in the tub, he finally stopped crying. Within a few minutes he was actually smiling and having fun. That is when I began using different salt baths regularly for Alex.

The main oils we used, and still use for the salt baths are Peace and Calming, Believe, Lavender, Lemon, and Thieves. All of our oils come from Young Living. I prefer Young Living oils because of their processing method that preserves the integrity and potency of the essential oil. You can find more info about Young Living oils at www.youngliving.com. You can also order from their website or through a distributor.

To make a salt bath:

- Mix one to two cups of Epsom Salt with four to six drops of essential oil.

- Pour mixture into warm bath.

- Mix until all salt has dissolved in bath.

BEDTIME

At this time, we had a strict routine to follow with Alex when it came to bedtime. It would take about 45 minutes to complete the routine. Most of our evenings were spent at home because we had to start his routine at 7:15 p.m. in order for him to be in bed by 8:00 p.m. so he would get the needed amount of sleep. His routine consisted of taking a bath, brushing teeth, reading a book, praying, singing a bedtime song, turning on a fan for white noise, and playing a radio with soft classical music. I also had to make sure his night lights were on and closet doors closed. On the weekends we were a little more lax with what time we began the routine so that we could enjoy an evening out, but we always did the routine.

BEDTIME ROUTINE

- Taking a bath
- Brushing teeth
- Reading a book
- Saying a prayer
- Singing a song
- Turning on white noise
- Playing soft classical music
- Turning on nightlights
- Closing closet doors

WORKING WITH THE SCHOOL

A follow up conference with the school was scheduled the next week to discuss the visit to the child psychologist. I shared what the child psychologist suggested. Alex's morning Montessori teacher and the director were okay with giving him some more guidelines and rules, as well as limiting his options on what he was allowed to work on for the day. However, his kindergarten teacher was not very enthusiastic about the changes. (He went to the kindergarten classroom for the afternoon.) Both his teachers kept a journal for the day so I knew if he had a "good day" or a "bad day" so Alex could have a negative consequence or a positive reward after school. The child psychologist suggested allowing him to play video games for about 20 minutes if he had a good day since we currently only allowed him to play on the weekends. When this was mentioned in the conference, his kindergarten teacher said if I did that it would make her job very difficult because she refused to give rewards for expected behavior. I informed the school and his teachers that I was going to follow the advice of a well respected doctor who specializes in these situations. His kindergarten teacher was also was very upset that she would have to take away some of Alex's decisions because that is NOT Montessori. However, it was agreed that both teachers would follow the new suggestions and limit his decision making on "work" he was allowed to choose from for the remainder of the year.

APPROACHING THE END OF KINDERGARTEN

Since there were only a few months left in the school year, we decided to keep him enrolled at that school. After the school made some corrections, and he was back on his neurotransmitter sprays, homeopathic remedies, and salt baths, his behavior improved drastically within a few weeks. He had no more incidents at school; however, his learning was still a concern. He continued to give little effort to his school work and didn't participate in many activities.

We had another conference with Alex's kindergarten teacher. She was very concerned that Alex wasn't grasping words and reading well. She then informed us that the other students were reading at a third grade level or at least a first grade level, but Alex was still struggling. I looked at this teacher and explained that I was not concerned about his reading in kindergarten. I told her that I never liked to read, and struggled with reading my whole life, but I was still able to go on and obtain two Bachelor's Degrees, and a Doctorate Degree. I guess now I can also add that I am able to write a book. She said, "Well, we do take a lot of pride in our kids reading well above average, and Alex is struggling." My husband almost jumped out of his seat and knocked her down. Thankfully, he has very good restraint.

REGULAR ACTIVITY

Another great step we did was enroll Alex in swimming lessons twice a week. He was extremely excited about swimming. Part of the problem with his behavior was the lack of exercise during the school day. That year, we had an unusually cold and long winter. The kids were unable to go outside to the playground for many months. The school didn't have a gym for the kids to run around in and play. Since Alex was a very active child, he absolutely needed to burn off some of his fuel. The standard swimming lessons were only once a week; and I knew he would need more. So, we enrolled him into two different sessions, one on Tuesday evenings and one on Thursday evenings. We chose swimming because it was indoors (winters are cold in the Midwest); he enjoyed it; and he was also learning a valuable skill. I suggest finding something your child is interested in and then do your best to support him. His teachers said they could tell a difference in his activity during the school day. He was a little more calm and had appropriate behavior. They also said that he was his best on Tuesdays and Thursdays. Hmmmm, I wonder why? Perhaps because he knew he had swimming those days and had something to look forward to doing. His teacher also told me he couldn't stop talking about swimming on those days.

That is when I realized the difference between the first year in this Montessori school and the second year. **It was the teacher.** I later discovered that the first set of teachers were let go because they would not adhere to the strict Montessori standards. Alex performed well the first year because he was able to have a combined Montessori and traditional school setting. The second year was strict Montessori, and he very quickly realized that he did not have to work his hardest. (Thank you, Ms. Felecia, for all your hard work the first year we were at the Montessori school.) I want to remind everyone that we chose a Montessori school because of how great they are at educating kids in all aspects of learning. It is a great teaching method and works wonders for many kids. Unfortunately, some of it just wasn't right for my son. It truly did help Alex master self skills and greatly improved his self esteem. For that I am forever thankful for the Montessori Method of teaching. However, each child is a unique individual and must be responded to as such. Parents should make the ultimate decision about what is best for their child.

This is the end of Alex's kindergarten year. We had great success with the neurotransmitter sprays, essential oils, and changing our parenting skills to fit Alex's need. The next chapter discusses the integration of specific essential oils for focusing and calming down behaviors. I also discuss the importance of a proper diet and growth mindset.

What did I learn in this chapter?

- Teachers play an extremely important role in a child's growth and behavior.
- A child's independence is important for good self-esteem.
- Proper food and diet are always important, especially for those children who are very active.
- Neurotransmitter support can help the brain function more efficiently and effectively.
- Therapeutic grade essential oils combined with Epsom Salt in a bath are a great aid for some behavioral problems.
- Daily exercise is a must for a kinesthetic learner or any child with some hyperactivity and/or focusing problems.

PART FIVE

A Wonderful Child

Currently Alex is six-and-a-half years old (I have to be certain to add the half otherwise he gets upset). He began first grade this year. At the beginning of the year he struggled a great deal with learning concepts and socializing skills. He attended a new, much larger private school that included kindergarten through sixth grade. His previous school was infant through kindergarten. As his teacher expressed to me, "He just had to trust me." It took a few months for him to become comfortable enough for him to trust his new teacher. He had a low self-esteem and after kindergarten he didn't seem to feel confident in his ability to do well in school.

The first week of school, the Dean of Students was able to have a chit-chat with him about his behavior. He was hitting some of his classmates on the playground and wasn't trying very hard in his schoolwork. Alex was able to express that he missed his older brother a lot and wanted him to come home. His older brother was gone on vacation with his dad for about ten days to visit his grandma. They are half brothers, so he wasn't able to go with him. The combination of that with starting a new, much larger school was enough for any kid to have a difficult first week.

I remember the first day of first grade at his new school. He walked into the building with a stern facial expression and walked straight to his classroom. I could tell my little man was extremely nervous. I asked him if he was okay, and he replied, "I'm a little nervous, but I can do it." I agreed with him and encouraged him as we walked down the hallway. I was proud that he was able to identify that he was nervous and still willing to give it a chance. We had been working on that quite a bit, using what we had learned about *Mindset*.

MINDSET

Alex was using a type of mindset. Since our boys were born we naturally would tell them that they were "so smart," not realizing that this statement was actually harming our sons more than helping them. Bonnie Davis, one of my patients, shared with me her work in an elementary school where the first grade teachers used *Mindset,* Carol Dweck's powerful tools of metacognition (Dweck, cited in Davis, p. 65). Metacognition is the ability to think about one's own thinking, and Dweck describes two kinds of metacognition or mindsets: a fixed mindset and a growth mindset. A fixed mindset is the belief that one's intelligence is fixed, and we either have it or not. A growth mindset is the belief that our mind is capable of "changing, growing, and continually learning" (p. 65). Fortunately, teachers and parents can explicitly teach mindset to children.

When children struggle with learning, it creates a sense of lowered confidence and learned helplessness. This is what we were beginning to see in Alex. With a fixed mindset, kids believe they are stuck with whatever they were born with intellectually. However, with a growth mindset, kids are encouraged to self-evaluate and try new things. A common growth mindset used in our house is "I know it's hard, but I will try." This new way of thinking and teaching our little Alex has been a huge success. As a parent, I had to acknowledge and understand that my child thinks differently than the majority of his classmates. He also doesn't learn as quickly as some of the other students. Once we started the phrase, "This is hard, but I will try," his entire attitude changed. He began to take more risks at home and with different sports. His teacher informed me today that his growth has been exponential in the classroom. He is now right where he needs to be at a first grade level. I love hearing him tell himself that wonderful phrase, "This is hard, but I will try."

Some other great growth mindset phrases are as follows:
I did it!
I can do this!
I will never give up.
I will try again.
Do your best.

Some fixed mindset phrases include:
I can't do it!
I give up.
I don't want to.
It's too hard.
I hate this.
I'll never know how.

We heard Alex say every single one of those fixed mindset statements up to first grade. It's heartbreaking as a parent. Now, we rarely hear any of those statements. He also is not allowed to say the phrase, "I can't do it." We encourage him in whatever it is he is trying.

FOCUS

Many of you are probably wondering if I do anything else with him during this school year, other than use the growth mindset. Well, yes I do. I continue to give him homeopathic remedies: Ignatia Amara and Belladonna; Acetylcholine neurotransmitter spray every morning (we give 2-3 sprays), and Salt Baths once a week or so. We have also added a few new things this year which really seem to help. One of them is Brain Power from Young Living Essential Oils. I really wasn't sure if I would notice anything with this one, but sure enough, his homework scores began increasing, and he began finishing his work more regularly at school. His teacher also informed me that he has been focusing really well at school. Is it just the oil or a combination of everything? I believe it's a combination. I don't think there is only one thing, or magic trick, that will correct all the symptoms associated with a hyperactive child who struggles with focusing and schoolwork.

ESSENTIAL OILS

Some of the essential oils from Young Living (www.youngliving.com) that I have found to help with increasing focus or have a calming effect are the following:

- Vetiver
- Brain Power
- Peace and Calming
- Lavender
- Valor
- Frankincense
- Focus

I recommend using Vetiver the evening before school (unless you home-school) as it has a very strong scent. It's also derived from a grass and can cause an allergic reaction to others nearby. I know this because it happened the first time I used it on Alex. I put a couple drops on the back of Alex neck and on the inside of his big toes in the morning. I dropped him off at school, and 30 minutes later I received a phone call from the headmaster that I needed to pick him up because his teacher was having a severe allergic reaction to his oil. They had to give her some Benadryl on site to relieve the symptoms. I discovered the oil is made from a grass. We only use the oil on the weekends now, which is unfortunate because it really does help.

Some other oils that can be helpful for symptoms of ADHD/ADD include the following:

- Cedarwood
- Harmony
- Gathering

- Clarity

I recommend diffusing the oil in the air nearby, especially during homework time. Before school (with the exception of Vetiver), I would put a couple drops on the base of the skull and the inside of the big toe on both feet. Both of these areas are reflexes for the brain. When applied to both areas at the same time, the oil affects the entire nervous system from head to toe.

PROTEIN

Another item we added was a high quality protein shake from Isagenix. At first, he didn't like them too much, but I just continued to give them to him and had him drink as much as he could. After about a week, he said they tasted okay. After two weeks, he actually liked them and was asking for them. I began giving him half the adult serving, one scoop instead of two of the Isagenix protein shake called Isalean Shake. Most people today don't consume enough protein, including kids. Alex has never really liked meat and doesn't eat enough beans and other high protein vegetables so I knew I needed to get some protein in him. The reason I chose the Isagenix shakes is because they have whey protein from New Zealand grass fed cows which is the best protein on the market. They also cold process the protein which allows the whey to remain undenatured for better absorption. The shakes also include a lot of digestive enzymes, prebiotics and probiotics, all of which are extremely important to have a healthy digestive tract. The shakes are also soy free and gluten free. I didn't want Alex having soy on a daily basis. Soy is estrogenic which can cause your body to think it's producing estrogen when in fact it's not. Gluten has the ability to create a large inflammatory reaction within your body so it's always a good precaution to avoid it when you can. Another reason adequate protein (amino acids) is important, specifically the amino acid called Tyrosine, is that it allows for proper brain function through the creation of dopamine and norepinephrine, which help a child's brain to stay alert and energized. I have since had some patients begin using it, including children who have ADHD, ADD, or Autism Spectrum Disorder.

I need to stress the importance of a high quality protein. A lot of "protein shakes" on the market are filled with by-products that can be harmful if used over a prolonged period of time. Isagenix has independent third party testing performed for quality standard. The protein shakes are also a meal replacement so it's filled with additional healthy calories, which is important for growing kids.

If you would like to order Isagenix, contact a

distributor or order from
www.thecenterfornaturalhealth.isagenix.com.

A lot of learning problems can come from a poor digestive system; therefore, it's important for your child to have a nutritionally sound diet.

WHOLE FOOD

Juice Plus is another great tool we use. Juice Plus is whole food nutrition that consists of over 30 vegetables, fruits, and grains. It's not a vitamin or mineral, rather complete whole food nutrition. We currently only give Alex what is called the Vineyard blend which includes a lot of different berries. Berries are filled with many antioxidants, and I wanted him to be able to expel toxins in his body effectively, which is one of the jobs antioxidants perform. Soon, we will start him on the vegetable blend and the fruit blend. It's also a nice treat for him since they come in the form of gummies. He thinks they are a treat. Juice Plus also has a Children's Health Study of over 150,000 participants that showed kids who take Juice Plus:

- Eat *less* fast food and *more* fruits and vegetables
- Drink *fewer* soft drinks and *more* water

- Visit the doctor *less* and attend school *more*

If you are interested in ordering Juice Plus, contact a distributor or order directly from www.at.juiceplus.com.

Combining the shakes, Juice Plus, and a healthy diet (for the most part) has helped tremendously with his attitude and behavior. My husband and I went out of town for a long weekend and left Alex with my parents. Alex had a really bad day at school. He was unfocused, talking out of turn, and disruptive in the class for a few days. I asked my mom what he had eaten for the weekend. Everything he had eaten seemed normal food for him until she said strawberry milk. Anytime Alex has too much processed, non-organic cow milk, I can tell he struggles with school a bit. Then, with the preservatives and artificial sweeteners you find in strawberry milk, it was way too much for him. I knew it would take about a week for it all to leave his system. It was actually a little less than a week because by Thursday he began getting his good remarks for behavior again. My mom now knows he is not allowed to have strawberry milk. We normally have him drink almond milk or coconut milk. Sometimes he is allowed organic cow milk.

I cannot stress enough the importance of a clean and healthy diet. Kids need to eat as many fresh fruits and vegetables as they can and really limit the amount of processed foods they eat. Eliminating all processed foods is ideal, but I understand how difficult it is in today's society.

CHANGING UP HIS ACTIVITY

We also signed him up for skating lessons this year, which have now turned into hockey lessons. He decided he was tired of swimming and wanted to try hockey. His older brother plays hockey, and he wants to be just like him (for now). We are letting him give it a go to see if it's something he truly wants. So far, he loves it and is excited every Tuesday and Saturday to go to hockey practice. It's also another good sport to burn off some of his energy. This year he has gym class everyday. I wish every school would incorporate gym class on a daily basis rather than two to three times per week. It makes such a big difference in young kids, especially challenging children.

Alex continues to do well in school this year. I'm excited to see how the rest of his future goes. Just like with anything, this is always going to be a work in progress. The same things that work now for him may not work in a few years. I'm continually looking at different approaches to see if one will work better than another.

I hope this book has helped you realize that there are great alternatives out there to help with your child. I understand that many are unable to afford to do everything, but even if you can find certain things that work, it's well worth the financial sacrifice. My husband and I have made financial sacrifices in order to afford the necessities needed for Alex. It's well worth it!

What did I learn in this chapter?

- A growth mindset is a great way to help foster young developing minds.
- Proper protein intake helps a child stay alert and energized.
- Proper amounts of fruits and vegetables are needed for healthy kids.
- Exercise, exercise, exercise!
- Continual positive support from parents and other adult authority figures is extremely important.
- Let kids try new things, and don't let them give up so easily when it's hard. This helps boost their self-esteem and become responsible adults.

PART SIX

Where We Are Now

Over the years, Alex has complained a lot about his legs hurting. There really is no reason for them to hurt. His pediatrician suggested they were growing pains. I even passed it off as growing pains, but then I realized kids aren't actually supposed to have growing pains. If their bodies have sufficient amounts of nutrients and minerals to help their bones grow, no pain is created. It wasn't until recently that I discovered a lot of Alex's leg pains are actually from an "allergic" reaction to the environment. This spring, Alex began complaining about his legs hurting again, so much so that he had difficulty walking. He hadn't complained about his legs hurting for many months. I would work on him through the use of chiropractic, essential oils, homeopathic remedies, etc., but nothing seemed to help for very long. After a few weeks of him complaining, he began to cough. That is when I thought of environmental allergies. I performed a NAET "boost" on him for his spring allergies. After this treatment, his legs began feeling better and his behavior improved. Environmental reactions don't necessarily have to be the classic watery eyes, runny nose, sneezing or coughing. Many times, they can present themselves in the sense of a foggy brain, difficulty thinking, body aches and pains, rashes, or strong negative emotional outbursts. This is often the case with Alex.

Not only can environmental allergies play a role in a child's behavior, but socioeconomic factors can also influence a child's behavior and ability to focus.

ADHD IN THE UNITED STATES AND FRANCE

Why does America have a higher rate of ADHD, at least 9%, compared to France, .05%? Marilyn Wedge, Ph.D., is a family therapist and author of three books as well as numerous journal articles in the field of family therapy. She states that *"instead of treating children's focusing and behavioral problems with drugs, French doctors prefer to look for the underlying issue that is causing the child distress — not in the child's brain but in the child's social context. They then choose to treat the underlying social context problem with psychotherapy or family counseling."* She goes on to state that *"the French holistic, psychosocial approach also allows for considering nutritional causes for ADHD-type symptoms -- specifically the fact that the behavior of some children is worsened after eating foods with artificial colors, certain preservatives, and/or allergens"(Wedge, 2012).*

French parents and physicians are well aware of the impact that dietary changes can help a child's problem. The strict focus on pharmaceutical treatment in the U.S. encourages physicians to ignore the impact dietary changes can have on a child's behavior.

The parenting styles between the United States and France are also very different. In the United States, American culture tends to give the children a lot of power in the household. In France the parents maintain control. American children are typically allowed to snack throughout the day, as opposed to French children. In France, there are four meals designated throughout the day, and the children need to wait for the scheduled meal. We began to narrow Alex's choices of meal times. He eats with the family at meal times but is also allowed one morning snack and one afternoon snack. This was difficult at first, but it became easier.

Everything takes time, and it's all about finding what works best for each person. Each person is very different, and not one thing fits all.

Everything is about balance, and I like to find the perfect balance for each individual. This is the road we are on, and I will continue to search for answers. Alex's behavior has been great for some time now, and his learning is continually improving. However, the end of the school year always provides a challenge with Alex's behavior and ability to focus.

As far as ADD/ADHD symptoms go, I believe we have found a very good balance of helping him maintain his focus while in school and at home. He is much calmer today than he was a year ago. I'm now working towards his overall health and keeping him healthy throughout his life by instilling good, positive healthy behaviors. Both my children rarely get sick, even when everyone around them is coming down with the flu or colds. That is primarily due to the fact that I keep their immune systems as strong as I can by feeding them healthy foods and catching any kind of illness at the beginning stage before it becomes symptomatic. Everyone in my family has a chiropractic adjustment regularly to maintain a healthy immune system.

Some of you might be wondering how adjusting the spine can help the immune system. A short answer is that our entire central nervous system is protected by the spine and skull. The nervous system stimulates the immune system; therefore, when an adjustment is made to the spine, it stimulates the immune system via the nervous system. Chiropractic adjustments can and should be done on everyone, no matter their age. My youngest patient was only three days old and my oldest was 83.

There are some children out there who truly need some help from medication. However, many children are able to be properly treated with alternative therapies and natural remedies. I would urge all of you to at least consider and try some of these natural alternatives to see if they help your child. Your son or daughter will thank you one day.

PART SEVEN

Additional Possible Medical Issues or Challenges

In this chapter, I will list and define possible medical issues or challenges that might be the cause of or contribute to certain behaviors. Not everyone will need everything written in this book, including Alex, but I have had success using a variety of the methods written here. These are additional medical scenarios to consider.

CANDIDA OVERGROWTH

Many people in our culture suffer from Candida overgrowth, more commonly known as yeast overgrowth. When people tend to think of a "yeast infection," they assume it only affects girls/women. This is often the case; however, it is possible to have Candida overgrowth in the intestines that affects both males and females alike. In fact, a lot of skin problems are due to Candida overgrowth or an inflammatory condition in the bowels. Whenever a patient comes into my office with the chief complaint of eczema or dry skin, I always look at food sensitivities and Candida. These two issues account for almost all of the eczema cases. According to the www.nationalcandidacenter.com:

"Candida Overgrowth (CO) symptoms are so numerous and seemingly unrelated that they can be confusing to both doctor and patient. The majority of people who have CO do not realize they have it until they become seriously ill. Why? Because Candida yeast not only steals nutrients from the food that you eat, it then poisons the tissues with waste material containing over 75 known toxins" (Vinikas, 1994).

The website has a great chart you can check to see if you or your child has a possibility of Candida overgrowth.

Candida overgrowth can be difficult to treat, depending on the severity. Alex developed thrush in his mouth shortly after birth. It took months for it to be healed. I was breast feeding at the time so it continued to pass from my nipple to his mouth. It was extremely uncomfortable for us both. However, having learned that a lot of ADD/ADHD symptoms can be due to yeast overgrowth in the body, this resonated with me. I decided to have Alex do a trial run of a Candida diet along with certain oral supplements. I am thankful my six-year-old is able to swallow any kind of pill, no matter the size, without any difficulty. My 10-year-old son struggles with swallowing pills and gets very perplexed that his younger brother has no difficulty. We tried it for a weekend just recently. I'm not going to lie...it was difficult. When you are trying to kill off Candida within the body, you have to avoid ALL FORMS OF SUGAR. This includes No grains, No dairy, No sugar, No yeast, No fruits, etc. He basically was left with vegetables and protein. I did cave and let him have an all beef hot dog (we don't normally eat hot dogs) without a bun. After just two days of this protocol along with certain supplements and herbs, he already showed improvement. I decided and informed Alex that during the summer we were going to do the protocol for a few weeks.

There is some astounding evidence that cancer is a fungus or can be caused by a fungus. Candida, or yeast, is a fungus. This is alarming since many individuals suffer from Candida Overgrowth. According to Mark A. Sircus, Ac., OMD:

"Cancer is a fungus, can be caused by a fungus, or is accompanied by late-stage fungal infections, and now the Mayo Clinic confirms this. They are not the first to say so though. Many, even from the official world of orthodox oncology, recognize the similarities of cancer and fungal infections, the decay that ties these two

together in a dance that all too often ends in miserable death" (Sircus, 2012).

The Mayo Clinic states that there is *"an emerging fungal infection of the gastrointestinal tract that mimics cancer and inflammatory bowel disease" (Cosway, 2012).* A lot of children, and adults for that matter, seem to have a lot of digestive issues. We can also bring Autism Spectrum Disorder into the conversation with regards to digestive issues.

Is it possible that a lot of the digestive problems associated with these conditions could be due to a fungal overgrowth in the bowels? There are many different effective strategies that help with fungal overgrowth. Of everything I treat in my office, yeast (fungus) is the most difficult. It is a multi-step process to eliminate, and it takes a lot of discipline on the patient's part. It requires prolonged treatment as well and can actually take up to two years for the body to completely get rid of the Candida overgrowth.

Candida has the ability to develop a resistance to herbs quickly within a couple days. Therefore, you need to alternate herbs. For example, one day use oregano, the next day use goldenseal, and on the third day, use thyme. Then start the rotation again. I highly recommend seeking out a doctor in your area that knows how to treat Candida and parasites as it can be difficult and tricky. Also, if you begin to kill off the Candida too quickly, you can get very ill.

PARASITES

Parasites are another possible issue in almost our entire population. According to Brenda Watson, ND, CT, a naturopathic doctor and colon therapist, states that *"Eighty-five percent of North Americans have at least one form of parasite. Some authorities believe that the true figure may be as high as 95 percent."* Some of the symptoms associated with a parasitic infection are the following:

- diarrhea and/or constipation
- gas, bloating, and cramps
- rectal itching
- persistent skin problems
- dark circles under the eyes
- lack of energy
- disturbed sleep
- muscle cramps or joint pain
- post-nasal drip

I haven't treated Alex for any parasitic infections yet. I will obtain a stool analysis to see if it shows anything; however, stool analysis only has about a 28% success rate.

Here is a list of some great remedies to help fight Candida and parasites:

- Oregano
- Thyme
- Pau D'Arco
- Candidase (great for yeast)
- Biocidin
- Baking soda
- Lavender Oil
- Tea Tree Oil
- Apple Cider Vinegar
- Garlic
- Coconut oil
- Excellent probiotic (high quality), (Yogurt does not contain enough probiotics to make a difference, and dairy feeds yeast.) I suggest Thorne Research and OrthoMolecular Products.
- Goldenseal
- Black Walnut oil

MTHFR

Many difficult and challenging children can actually have a genetic "mutation" that doesn't allow their bodies to eliminate toxins efficiently or allow proper reproduction of new cells. This mutation is called MTHFR. MTHFR stands for methylene tetrahydrofolate reductase. It is an enzyme designed to break down folate (B-9) and vitamin B-12 (cyanocobalamin) into a usable form in our bodies. It converts an amino acid called homocysteine into another amino acid called methionine. This is part of the methylation cycle. Methylation is extremely important for detoxification, immune support, mood balance, controlling inflammation, energy production, and it helps repair our DNA on a daily basis. It plays an important role in getting toxins out of the body.

A lot of children who have ADHD have a mutation in this gene, which decreases its ability to methylate. A study was published in *The International Journal of Medical Sciences* that showed a significant difference in the A1298C MTHFR gene mutation between the control group and the ADHD participants in areas of inattentiveness, hyperactivity/impulsivity. However, there were no statistically significant differences with the C677T MTHFR. It also found that *"eight of nine girls from the ADHD group were found to have A1298C mutation, but no statistical difference was found when compared with the control group"* (Gokcen C, Kocak N, Pekgor A).

Dr. Amy Yasko and Dr. Ben Lynch are the two leading authorities on MTHFR and methylation. Dr. Yasko has a protocol when dealing with methylation issues. I decided not to take her route as it requires a lot of supplementation. It requires too many vitamins for Alex to take at one time. I am opting to have testing done by a saliva test from Dr. Lynch's recommendation at www.23andme.com. The results from www.23andme.com come in raw data form so we will input the raw data into another website, www.geneticgenie.com. That will give us a good assessment if Alex has any issues with his methylation pathway. I recommend every child with ADD/ADHD have this testing done. You can order the test yourself on those websites. The test is easy and currently costs $99. Someone who has an MTHFR mutation needs to avoid as many chemicals and toxins as one can from daily life as their body is unable to filter the toxins out easily. I suggest you look at Dr. Lynch's website at www.MTHFR.net for some guidance.

I, myself, have a double mutation (one from my mom and one from my dad). My husband hasn't been tested, but it's likely he has a mutation since his oldest son, my stepson, has mild autism. It's estimated that 98% of children with autism have an MTHFR mutation as suggested by a study published in the *Journal of American Physicians and Surgeons*. It noted that *"only 2% of children with ASD in our study presented without at least one polymorphism in the MTHFR gene"* (Boris M, Goldblatt A, Galanko J, James J). Therefore, it's extremely likely that Alex has some form of mutation on his MTHFR gene. This is another reason we chose to start with the Vineyard blend from Juice Plus. Berries naturally have the already converted form of folate so Alex's body is able to use it appropriately. It's also advised to decrease your intake of folic acid, which is the synthetic form of folate, because people with MTHFR mutations have a decreased ability to neutralize the folic acid. Folic acid that has not been neutralized can lead to many health problems. These individuals **NEED to eat whole fresh food**. Avoid processed foods as much as you can. This is another reason we are getting ready to add the vegetable blend and fruit blend to Alex's daily routine from Juice Plus because it's whole food.

FRESH FRUITS AND VEGETABLES

We also began a Tower Garden from Juice Plus this year to help increase his daily intake of fresh organic vegetables and fruits. In my experience, kids who are able to help plant and cultivate food are more likely to try it and begin to enjoy eating the food they help grow. This is the route I chose because I don't have a "green thumb." I also don't have a lot of time to work on a traditional garden. The Tower Garden is aeroponic (grows without dirt), uses 10% of the water and space of a regular garden, and has less problems with insects. For more information on Tower Gardens, visit www.at.juiceplus.com. However, if you are great with gardens and enjoy gardening, that is also a great route. Make sure you don't use any pesticides, herbicides, or fungicides on your garden. MTHFR mutations are unable to eliminate those effectively.

What did I learn in this chapter?

- Candida (yeast) overgrowth is a health problem we need to begin considering on many levels.
- Hidden, sub-clinical parasitic infections can create a lot of health issues, including brain fog and a leaky gut.
- Food and parenting does indeed play a role in ADD/ADHD.
- There is a correlation between MTHFR mutations and ADHD.

ORDERING INFORMATION

I am providing a list of places you can order the items listed in the book for easy reference.

Essential Oils: www.youngliving.com.

Genetic Testing: First at www.23andme.com, then follow up at www.geneticgenie.com after results are received. Follow instructions for downloading results.

Homeopathic Remedies: www.1800homeopathy.com

Isagenix Protein Shakes and Bars: www.thecenterfornaturalhealth.isagenix.com or from a local distributor.

Juice Plus: www.at.juiceplus.com or from a local distributor.

MTHFR information: www.MTHFR.net.

Tower Garden: www.at.juiceplus.com or from a local distributor.

Vitamins: Quality vitamins can be ordered from www.amazon.com or from www.vitacost.com. Some of the brands I prefer are:
- Apex Energetics
- Biotics Research
- Metagenics
- Thorne Research

TIMELINES

The timeline below depicts the course I took with Alex from beginning to present.

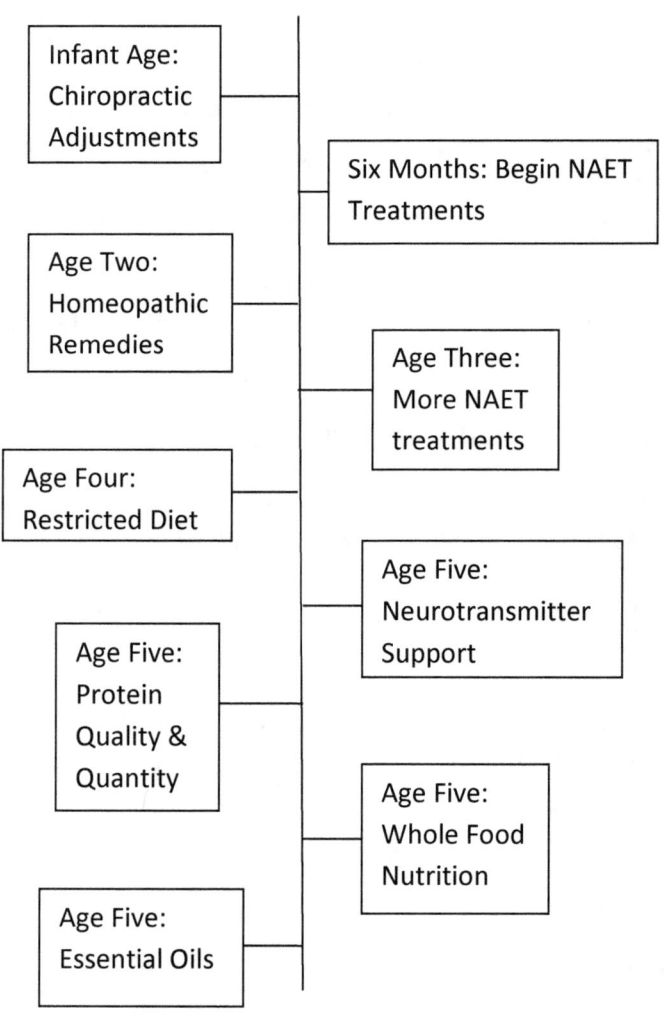

Infant Age: Chiropractic Adjustments

Six Months: Begin NAET Treatments

Age Two: Homeopathic Remedies

Age Three: More NAET treatments

Age Four: Restricted Diet

Age Five: Neurotransmitter Support

Age Five: Protein Quality & Quantity

Age Five: Whole Food Nutrition

Age Five: Essential Oils

The timeline below depicts the course I recommend others to try before adding the next therapy. I recommend starting as young as possible. However, it's never too late to begin. Whatever your child's age, you can begin treatment now.

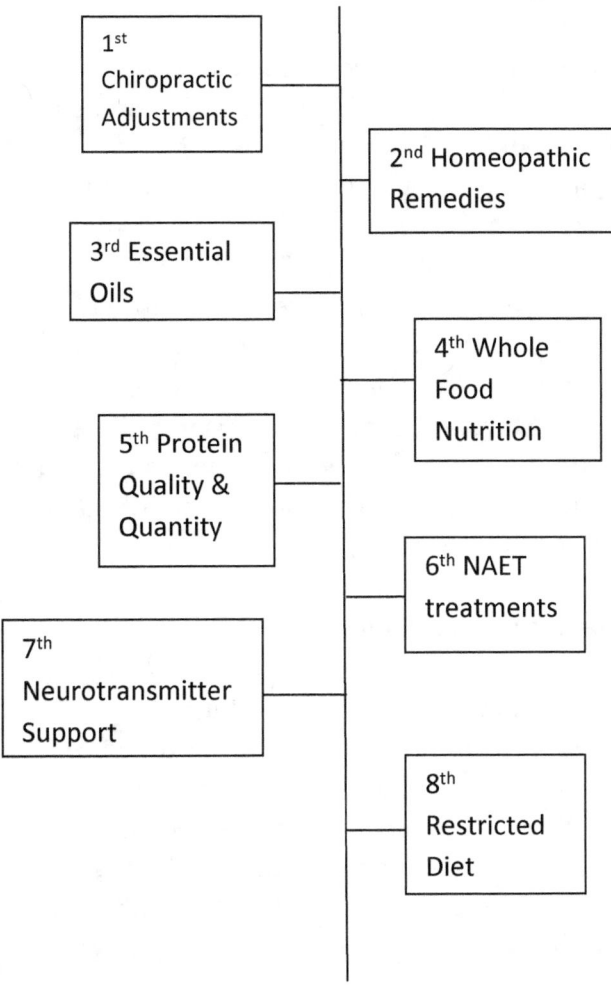

1st Chiropractic Adjustments

2nd Homeopathic Remedies

3rd Essential Oils

4th Whole Food Nutrition

5th Protein Quality & Quantity

6th NAET treatments

7th Neurotransmitter Support

8th Restricted Diet

APPENDIX A

HOMEOPATHIC REMEDY RESEARCH

What is homeopathy?

Homeopathy traces its roots back to Samuel Hahnemann (1755-1843). Hahnemann graduated medical school in 1779 and began his first homeopathy experiments in 1790. He began his journey of finding a better way to help patients with the principles of "similars" or "like cures like." The idea of "like cures like" can be traced back to Hippocrates and Paracelsus. It was also used by many cultures, including Native Americans, Mayans, Chinese, and Asian Indians, but Hahnemann is the one who developed it into a systematic medical science which is used in a large part of the world today.

Where is homeopathy used?

The U.S. experienced a disinterest in homeopathy in the 20th century, but the practice of it remained very active and alive in the rest of the world, including countries in Europe and Asia. However, homeopathy has begun to make a re-emergence in the U.S. In the 1970's, there were 50-100 physicians who specialized in homeopathy;

today there are over 1,000 health professionals utilizing the benefits of homeopathy. The National Center for Homeopathy, located in Virginia, states that 230 million dollars were spent by Americans on homeopathic remedies in 1996 and sales are rapidly rising at 12-15% each year. Almost all pharmacies in France sell homeopathic remedies and medicines. There is also a very strong use of homeopathy in Russia, Switzerland, Netherlands, Italy, South America, India, Mexico, Germany, and England. In fact, the royal family of Great Britain has been under homeopathic care since the 1830's (Ullman, 1991).

Philosophy of Homeopathy

The philosophy of homeopathy is based on "like treating like." Hahnemann introduced the idea of "miasms." A miasm is a "body memory" of something that occurred. Homeopaths believe that each disease is attributed with a specific miasm that creates a local symptom such as a rash to develop when triggered by a certain stimuli. Hahnemann stated that if a disease was treated with a medication, the disease would be driven deeper into the body. This is known as suppression. Homeopathic practitioners believe that the suppression of a disease will eventually lead to the internal organs becoming diseased. They also believe all diseases have a chronic underlying cause that must be treated by addressing the symptoms (not opposing the symptoms). The miasm will still remain and must be corrected in order to eliminate the disturbance being caused by a vital force.

How does homeopathy work?

Homeopathy is based on "resonance" which is based on the principles of physics. Every plant, herb, minerals, etc., has its own specific vibrational field that can exert a healing effect on the body. This energy field can be "potentiated," or amplified, by a series of dilutions and vigorous shaking. In order for healing to occur, the correct vibrational resonance must be used. For instance, too much cold in the intestines (constipation) needs to be treated with the correct homeopathic remedy that causes constipation. The person must be hypersensitive to the remedy, or they will not notice any difference. Homeopathic remedies are diluted concentrations of the actual substance. For example, Belladonna comes from the belladonna plant and is used in a highly diluted quantity. The diluted substances have been effective in treating many ailments.

APPENDIX B
An open letter and quoted from NAET

NAET
(Nambudripad Allergy Elimination Technique)

What are Nambudripad's Allergy Elimination Techniques?

Overview

NAET® was discovered by Dr. Devi S. Nambudripad in November of 1983. Nambudripad's Allergy Elimination Techniques, also known as NAET, are a non-invasive, drug free, natural solution to alleviate allergies of all types and intensities using a blend of selective energy balancing, testing and treatment procedures from acupuncture/acupressure, allopathy, chiropractic, nutritional, and kinesiological disciplines of medicine.

One allergen is treated at a time. If you are not severely immune deficient, you may need just one treatment to desensitize one allergen. A person with mild to a moderate number of allergies may need 15-20 office visits to desensitize 15-20 food and environmental allergens.

Basic essential nutrients are treated during the

first few visits. Chemicals, environmental allergens, vaccinations, immunizations, etc., are treated after completing about ten basic essential nutrients. NAET can successfully alleviate adverse reactions to egg, milk, peanuts, penicillin, aspirin, mushrooms, shellfish, latex, grass, ragweed, flowers, perfume, animal dander, animal epithelial, make-up, chemicals, cigarette smoke, pathogens, heat, cold, and other environmental agents. It may take several office visits to desensitize a severe allergen.

NAET is available all over the world. Over 12,000 licensed medical practitioners have been trained in NAET procedures and are practicing world-wide. To help you find a NAET specialist, the names of the trained practitioners have been listed on our website under the "Find a Practitioner" section. We ask that you browse the NAET website for more information on NAET and use our practitioner locator to find a NAET practitioner near you.

All NAET practitioners in the practitioner locator have been trained by Dr. Nambudripad, but it is not possible for us to track each practitioner's performance. Please understand that these trained NAET practitioners are independent medical practitioners, some may be doing various treatment procedures other than NAET.

It is your job to find the right practitioner for your treatment. Please read the open letter by Dr. Nambudripad, to become well informed before you make an appointment with a NAET practitioner.

Allopathy & Western Sciences

Knowledge of the brain, cranial nerves, spinal nerves and autonomic nervous system from Western medicine enlightens us about the body's efficient multilevel communication network. Through this network of nerves, vital energy circulates through the body carrying negative and positive messages from the brain to each and every cell in the body and back to the brain. Knowledge of the nervous system, its origin, travel pathway, the organs and tissues that will benefit from its nerve energy supplies (target organs and tissues) and its destination, helps us to understand the energy distribution of particular spinal nerves that emerge from the 31 pairs of spinal nerve roots.

Kinesiology

Kinesiology is the art and science of movement of the human body. Kinesiology is used in NAET to compare the strength and weakness of any muscle (also known as neuromuscular sensitivity testing (NST)) of the body in the presence and absence of any substance. A measured weakness in the presence of a substance is due to the effect of an allergy to the item the person is touching. This simple method can be used to detect your allergens.

Chiropractic

Chiropractic principles help us to detect the nerve energy blockage in a specific nerve energy pathway by detecting and isolating the exact nerve root being pinched. The exact vertebral level in relation to the pinched spinal nerve root helps us to trace the travel route, the destination and the target organs of that particular energy pathway. D.D. Palmer, considered the "Father of Chiropractic," said, "Too much or too little energy is disease." A pinched nerve can cause disturbance in the energy flow. Chiropractic medicine postulates that a pinched nerve or any such disturbance in the energy flow can cause disease, revealing the importance of maintaining an uninterrupted flow of nerve energy. A pinched nerve or an obstruction in the energy flow is often the result of an allergy. Spinal manipulation at the specific vertebral level of the pinched nerve can relieve the obstruction of the energy flow and help the body to arrive at a state of homeostasis.

Acupuncture / Oriental Medicine

Yin-Yang theory from Oriental medical principles teaches the importance of maintaining homeostasis in the body. According to Oriental medical principles, "When the body is in perfect balance, no disease is possible." Any disturbance in the homeostasis can cause disease. Any allergen capable of producing a weakening muscular effect in the body can cause disturbance in homeostasis. Hence, diseases can be prevented and cured by maintaining homeostasis. According to acupuncture theory, acupuncture and/or acupressure at certain acupuncture points is capable of bringing the body to a state of homeostasis by removing the energy blockages from the energy pathways known as meridians. When the blockages are removed, energy can flow freely through the energy meridians, thus bringing the body in perfect balance.

Nutrition

You are what you eat! The secret to good health is achieved through right nutrition. What is right nutrition? And how do you get it? When you can eat nutritious foods without discomfort and assimilate their nutrients, that food is said to be the right food. When you get indigestion, bloating, or other digestive troubles upon eating the food, that food is not helping you function normally. This is due to an allergy to the food. Different foods react differently in different people. What is food for some may be poison for others. You've probably heard the expression, "One man's meat is another man's poison." So it is very important to clear the allergy to the nutrients. Allergic people can tolerate food that is low in nutrition better than nutritious food. But upon clearing the allergy, you should try to eat more wholesome, nutritious foods. You should avoid refined, bleached food that is devoid of nutrients. Many people who are feeling poorly due to undiagnosed food allergies may take vitamins or other supplements to increase their vitality after they get treated for the specific allergy. If they happen to be allergic to the nutritional supplements they are taking, this can actually make them feel worse. Only after clearing those allergies can their bodies properly assimilate them. So nutritional assessment should be done periodically, and, if needed, appropriate supplements should be taken to receive faster results.

*Appendix B is reprinted from http://www.naet.com/Patients/whatsnaet.aspx with written permission from Devi Nambudripad, M.D., D.C. Further information and practitioner location can be found at www.naet.com or www.naetautismtreatmentcenter.com.

APPENDIX C

ANTIOXIDANTS

Antioxidants are like an excellent housekeeper; "mopping up free radicals before they get a chance to harm your body." *

Oxidation — A Natural Chemical Reaction

To understand how antioxidants work, you must first understand oxidation. We have all seen a copper penny turn green and a fender on a car rust. We have also all seen how, after biting into an apple, the pulp turns from white to brown when the apple is left exposed to the air for too long. This happens because oxygen reacts with the pulp, causing it to discolor. When oxygen interacts with substances, from metals to living tissue, this is called oxidation.

Oxygen — The Dual-Edged Sword

We depend on oxygen for our survival, but oxygen is also a forceful molecule that is capable of reacting negatively with other molecules. The discoloration of the apple is an example of the wear and tear that happens when oxygen reacts with living molecules. Without some type of protection against the oxygen in the air, the pulp of the apple is assaulted by it. While oxygen is essential for health, it is also capable of producing molecules called oxygen "free radicals." When you don't have enough "antioxidant defense mechanisms" against these free radicals, your health can be compromised in much the same manner as what causes an apple to discolor.

Free Radicals vs. Antioxidants — Like a "Mini-War"

Antioxidants can be enzymes, vitamins, bio-flavonoids, minerals, and other substances that can provide protection from the damaging effects of free radicals. Imagine a "mini-war" in which your body is the battlefield. Inside you, the attacking forces (the free radicals) are aggressively fighting the protective forces (the antioxidants). Over 100 adverse health conditions have been associated with excessive free-radical activity. Free radicals affect every part of your body from your eyes and skin to your circulatory system and immune system, even to the way your body recovers from a wound.

Kinds of Antioxidants — Targeted Protection

Antioxidants have a broad activity range within

all cells of the body. Certain antioxidant nutrients and botanicals appear to have a particular affinity for certain bodily tissues. Some types of antioxidants and their generalized functions are the following:

- **Alpha-Lipoic acid** – is an antioxidant in both fat-soluble and water-soluble environments so it can benefit all body tissues, although it has a special affinity for the liver and nerves.
- **Bilberry** – has a particular affinity for the eyes, especially the retina.
- **Coenzyme Q10** – has a particular affinity for the energy-producing powerhouses (mitochondria) in every cell of the body.
- **Curcumin** – the primary flavonoid in the spice turmeric has special affinities for the liver, GI tract, and musculoskeletal system.
- **Ginkgo Biloba** – contains important antioxidant flavonoids with particular affinity for the brain and circulatory system.
- **Glutathione** – is produced in the body and has special importance for the liver and brain.
- **Grape seed extract** – sometimes referred to as OPCs has a special affinity for the blood vessels and collagen support.

- **Green tea extract** – provides special antioxidant protection for the skin from ultraviolet radiation and helps with normal cell formation.
- **Milk thistle extract** – has a special affinity for the liver.
- **Quercetin** – a flavonoid found in hundreds of fruits, vegetables, and other plants, has particular affinity for the mucus membranes of the respiratory tract.
- **Selenium** – works with glutathione in the body and protects cell membranes from oxidation.
- **Vitamin C** – is an antioxidant in water-soluble environments in the body such as the cell interior.
- **Vitamin E** – an antioxidant in fat-soluble environments in the body such as the cell membrane, prevents oxidation of cholesterol for cardiovascular support.
- **Zinc** – is a cofactor for the antioxidant superoxide dismutase (SOD) that is produced in the body and also helps prevent oxidative damage from too much iron.

Obtaining Antioxidants — The Natural Way

Antioxidants are plentiful in such common vitamins as vitamin A, ascorbic acid or vitamin C, vitamin E, and selenium. Research confirms that a balanced diet rich in whole-grain cereals, nuts, seeds, fruits, and vegetables can provide the essential vitamins, minerals, antioxidants, and other nutrients that promote the good health of a number of the body's systems, including cardiovascular health, immune health, connective tissue health, cognitive health, and gingival health.

According to the U.S. Department of Agriculture, most Americans don't consume the "five-a-day recommended servings of fruits and vegetables." To ensure you are providing your body with adequate protection from free-radical damage, it makes sense to supplement your diet with a range of vitamin, mineral, and herbal antioxidants.*

Other Things to Consider — Sunscreen on the Inside

Avoid processed foods as much as possible. Try to eat plenty of fresh, organic whole foods, especially a variety of richly colored fresh fruits and vegetables. Sweet or purple potatoes, carrots, bell peppers, spinach, cantaloupe, blueberries, raspberries, and mangoes are great sources of antioxidants. Plants make antioxidants to protect themselves from the sun's ultraviolet radiation, so when we eat colorful fruits and vegetables those same pigments (or colorings) can protect us, too. Typically speaking, the deeper and richer the color of a fruit or vegetable, the more potent are its antioxidant properties.

Make an effort to reduce or eliminate exposure to toxic chemicals (e.g., household cleaners, petrochemicals, etc.). Take high quality, pure dietary supplements recommended by your health-care practitioner.

References and Resources

Catalá-López, Ferrán et al. *"The Pharmacological and Non-Pharmacological Treatment of Attention Deficit Hyperactivity Disorder in Children and Adolescents: Protocol for a Systematic Review and Network Meta-Analysis of Randomized Controlled Trials."* Systematic Reviews 4 (2015): 19. PMC. Web. 4 Apr. 2015.

Chellappa SL, Steiner R, Blattner P, Oelhafen P, Götz T, et al. (2011) *Non-Visual Effects of Light on Melatonin, Alertness and Cognitive Performance: Can Blue-Enriched Light Keep Us Alert?* PLoS ONE 6(1): e16429. doi:10.1371/journal.pone.0016429

Cosway, L. (2012). *Mayo Clinic Reports Emerging Fungal Infection in Southwest That Mimics Cancer.* Accessed at www.newsnetwork.mayoclinic.org/discussion/mayo-clinic-reports-emerging-fungal-infection-in-southwest-that-mimics-cancer/?_ga=1.107273410.1910609300.1422820781 on February 12, 2015.

Davis, Bonnie M. (2014). *Cultural Literacy for the Common Core: Six Steps to Powerful, Practical Instruction for All Learners.* Bloomington, IN: Solution Tree Press.

Dweck, Carol S. (2006). *Mindset: The New Psychology of Success.* New York: Random House.

Ferber, Richard. (2006). *Solve Your Child's Sleep Problems.* (pp. 10-11). New York: Fireside Book.

Frei, H, Everts R, von Ammon K, Kaufmann F, Walther D, Hsu-Schmitz SF, Collenberg M, Fuhrer K, Hassink R, Steinlin M, Thurneysen A. *Homeopathic treatment of children with attention deficit hyperactivity disorder: a randomised, double blind, placebo controlled crossover trial.* Eur J Pediatr., July 27,2005, 164:758-767.

Frei, H, and Thurneysen, A. *Treatment for Hyperactive Children: Homeopathy and Methylphenidate Compared in a Family Setting.* British Homeopathic Journal, October 2001, 90:183-188.

Hattie, J. (2009). *Visible Learning: A Synthesis of over 800 Meta-Analyses relating to Achievement* (pp. 194-199). New York, NY: Routledge.

Hattie, J. and Yates, G.C.R. (2014). *Visible Learning and the Science of How We Learn* (pp. 176-183). New York, NY: Routledge.

Linksman, R. (1999). *The Fine Line Between ADHD and Kinesthetic Learners.* Accessed at http://latitudes.org/the-fine-line-between-adhd-and-kinesthetic-learners on April 4, 2015.

Nambudri pad, D. (2014). *What are Nambudripad Allergy Elimination Techniques?* Accessed at www.naet.com/Patients/whatsnaet.aspx on

February 12, 2015.

Sircus, M. (2012). *Baking Soda, Cancer, and Fungus.* Accessed at www.naturalnews.com on February 13, 2015.

Ullman, D. (1991*). Discovering Homeopathy: Medicine for the 21st Century.* Berkeley, CA: North Atlantic Books.

Vinikas, B. (1994). *National Candida Center Self Exam.* Accessed at www.nationalcandidacenter.com/candida-self-exams on January 29, 2015.

Watson, B. (2005). *Parasite Cleansing.* Accessed at www.alive.com/articles/view/19034/parasite_cleansing on February 4, 2015.

Wedge, M. (2012). *Why French Kids Don't Have ADHD.* Accessed at www.psychologytoday.com/blog/suffer-the-children/201203/why-french-kids-dont-have-adhd on February 14, 2015.

www.ingramcontent.com/pod-product-compliance
Lightning Source LLC
Chambersburg PA
CBHW060420290526
45791CB00002B/840